VERY
Blueberry

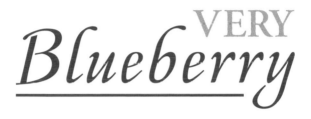

VERY
Blueberry

Jennifer Trainer Thompson

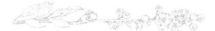

CELESTIAL ARTS
Berkeley | Toronto

*A special thanks to Linda Stripp and Jody Fijal
for their help with this book.*

Copyright © 2005 by Jennifer Trainer Thompson

CA

Celestial Arts
P.O. Box 7123
Berkeley, California 94707
www.tenspeed.com

Distributed in Australia by Simon and Schuster Australia, in Canada by Ten Speed Press Canada, in New Zealand by Southern Publishers Group, in South Africa by Real Books, and in the United Kingdom and Europe by Airlift Book Company.

Cover and text design by Chloe Rawlins

Library of Congress Cataloging-in-Publication Data
Thompson, Jennifer Trainer.
  Very blueberry / Jennifer Trainer Thompson.
    p. cm.
  Summary: "More than 50 recipes for entrees, salads, desserts, and gifts featuring blueberries"
  ISBN-10: 1-58761-193-7 (pbk.)
  ISBN-13: 978-1-58761-193-3 (pbk.)
  1. Cookery (Blueberries) I. Title.

TX813.B5T48 2005
  641.6'4737—dc22   2004021574

Printed in Singapore
First printing, 2005

3 4 5 6 7 8 9 10—09 08 07 06

Contents

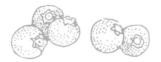

Introduction

I have a big heart for these little books. I remember picking blueberries as a kid in Maine in August (and reading *Blueberries for Sal* by Robert McCloskey all winter), and more recently, canoeing in bathing suits out to Blueberry Island on top of Mt. Riga with my son. We used old Folgers coffee cans to collect wild blueberries, the *kerplink kerplunk* of the first few berries eventually giving way to a softer *pfffftt* as we neared the top. That was assuming we didn't eat more than we picked of these sun-warmed indigo marvels that look like a clear summer sky and are so much tastier than their insipid, marble-size cousins sold in chain grocery stores.

Like chiles, wild berries vary in taste from bush to bush and range in flavor from sweet to puckery-tart. With birds transporting them far afield, you'll come across wild blueberries growing on the Appalachian Trail, in Quebec fields, on Maine mountaintops, and in the marshes of Fire Island. They've grown wild for thousands of years. Native Americans were wise enough to use them way back when as a root tea poultice to help women relax during childbirth. Low-bush blueberry bushes (which grow to a foot or two high) thrive in glacial soils and in the higher elevations of Canada and New England. The berries are small and hard to pick but are well worth it. Bakers love them because they hold their shape. It may take an hour of backbreaking work to pick enough for a pie, but the pie will be gorgeous when you cut into it and see those glistening blue pearls. High-bush blueberry bushes can reach shoulder height and higher, and are mostly cultivated (though we have some wild ones atop Mt. Riga). Their fruit can be sweeter than low-bush berries.

Cousin to the azalea and rhododendron, blueberries like acidic soil and have a beautiful red foliage in the fall. The best time to plant blueberry bushes is in spring. And keep in mind, they like company. I have always been amused that you get a better yield if you plant several bushes of different varieties together, allowing the plants to cross-pollinate. (I thought this a charming feature and once made a wedding gift of a pair of blueberry bushes.) A mature bush will yield up to twenty pounds of berries during a single harvest, and a harvest typically lasts about four weeks.

Blueberry bushes look good (if you can beat the bears and birds to the berries), and the berries are incredibly good for you. Their antioxidants may prevent some serious health problems from Alzheimer's and Parkinson's to cancer, diabetes, circulation problems, and urinary tract infections. A recent study also indicates that they may help prevent heart disease. A research chemist in Mississippi recently determined that a certain compound found in blueberries (called pterostilbene) may possibly lower cholesterol as well as drugs on the market do. Scientists haven't moved yet beyond the early testing phase, nor have they proposed how many blueberries one would have to eat, but it does seem clear: blueberries can help fight a multitude of ailments. Moreover, they are rich in fiber and vitamin C (a half cup is equivalent to one thousand milligrams of vitamin C).

To enjoy berries year-round, simply place them, unwashed, in a single layer on a baking sheet and freeze them. Remove the pan from the freezer, place the berries in sealed plastic bags, and return them to the freezer for up to six months.

Never wash berries—fresh, dried, or frozen—until you're about to serve them or use them to brighten muffins or pancakes, enliven rice and salad, or add color to desserts. Swirled into your pancake batter in January, they will remind you of that hot August afternoon you picked the perfect blue ball and popped it into your mouth while it was still warm from the sun.

Breakfast and Snacks

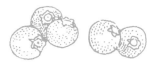

Blueberry-Almond Danish Coffee Cake

Blueberries mingle deliciously with almonds in this rich coffee cake. It's an unforgettable start to the day.

Topping

¾ cup packed light brown sugar

¼ cup granulated sugar

⅔ cup all-purpose flour

1 teaspoon ground cinnamon

6 tablespoons salted butter, cold, cut into small pieces

½ cup chopped almonds

Filling

12 ounces light or regular cream cheese,
   at room temperature

⅓ cup sugar

1 egg

1 tablespoon heavy whipping cream

1 teaspoon pure almond extract

(continued)

Cake

4 cups all-purpose flour

1 tablespoon plus 1 teaspoon baking powder

½ teaspoon salt

½ cup salted butter, at room temperature

1¼ cups sugar

2 eggs

1½ teaspoons pure vanilla extract

1½ teaspoons pure almond extract

1 cup milk

3 cups fresh or thawed frozen blueberries

To make the topping, combine the brown sugar, granulated sugar, flour, and cinnamon in a small bowl. Using a pastry blender or your fingers, cut in the butter until the mixture is crumbly. Stir in the almonds and set aside.

To make the filling, in the bowl of an electric mixer, beat the cream cheese and sugar on medium-high, until fluffy. Add the egg, cream, and almond extract, and beat until fully incorporated, 1 to 2 minutes. Set aside.

To make the cake, preheat the oven to 375°F. Butter a 9 by 13-inch glass pan. Combine the flour, baking powder, and salt in a small bowl. Beat the butter in large bowl on medium-high, until creamy. Add the sugar and continue to beat until fluffy. Beat in the eggs, vanilla extract, and almond extract, and continue to beat until fluffy and light. Add the flour mixture alternately with the milk, beating well after each addition.

Spread half of the batter in the prepared pan. Spread the cream cheese filling in a layer over the batter. Sprinkle the blueberries in an even layer over the filling. Drop the remaining batter in spoonfuls over the top, and spread evenly; do not mix the layers. Top with the sugar-almond mixture. Place in the oven and bake for 1 hour and 5 minutes, or until deep golden brown. Let the cake cool in the pan completely before cutting.

Serves 12 to 16

Blueberry-Banana Bread

This is a good use for summer blueberries frozen and saved for winter.

2 cups all-purpose flour
½ cup granulated sugar
¼ cup brown sugar
1½ teaspoons baking powder
1 teaspoon baking soda
1 teaspoon salt
2 eggs, beaten
1 teaspoon pure vanilla extract
3 tablespoons unsalted butter, melted
3 bananas, mashed (about 1½ cups)
1½ cups fresh or frozen blueberries

Preheat the oven to 350°F. Coat a 3 by 8-inch metal loaf pan with nonstick cooking spray. (Note: Ovenproof glass conducts heat more than metal does, so if you're using a glass rather than a metal loaf pan, decrease the oven temperature by 25 degrees.)

In a large bowl, sift together the flour, granulated sugar, brown sugar, baking powder, baking soda, and salt. In a separate bowl, combine the eggs, vanilla, butter, and bananas and mix well. Make a well in the center of the dry ingredients. Add the liquid ingredients all at once. Stir only enough to moisten. Add the blueberries and gently fold in. Turn into the prepared loaf pan. Place in the oven and bake for 1 hour and 30 minutes, or until top is golden-brown. Bread is done when a toothpick inserted into the center of the loaf comes out clean. Cool in the pan for 5 minutes, then transfer to a cooling rack. Serve warm. To store bread, wrap in aluminum foil or plastic wrap and freeze for up to 2 months.

Makes 1 loaf

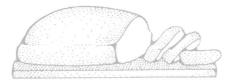

Blueberry-Ginger Scones

Dried blueberries are available in gourmet stores or high-end super-markets. Scones are best served warm from the oven with butter or jam. Traditionally, they are served with clotted cream or whipped cream.

2 cups all-purpose flour
1 teaspoon salt
2 tablespoons sugar
1 teaspoon baking soda
1 teaspoon baking powder
¼ cup crystallized ginger, chopped
¼ cup dried blueberries
½ cup cold unsalted butter, diced
½ cup plus 1 tablespoon heavy whipping cream
1 egg, lightly beaten

Preheat the oven to 350°F. In the bowl of a food processor fitted with the metal blade, combine the flour, salt, sugar, baking soda, baking powder, ginger, and blueberries and pulse to mix. Add the butter and pulse until the mixture looks like coarse cornmeal. Transfer to a bowl. Add the ½ cup heavy cream and stir until the dough comes together, taking care not to overmix. Turn the dough out onto a lightly floured work surface and knead gently, folding about 10 times, or until the dough holds together and its consistency is smooth. Gather the dough into a ball and flatten into a 6-inch disk. Cut the disk into 8 wedges. Place the wedges 2 inches apart on an ungreased baking sheet. In a small bowl, combine the remaining 1 tablespoon of heavy cream with the egg and beat lightly. Brush the scones with the egg wash. Place in the oven and bake for 20 minutes, or until golden. Cool 5 minutes, then transfer to wire cooling rack to cool. Best served immediately.

Makes 8 scones

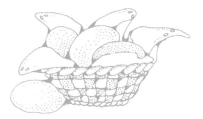

Blueberry Corn Pancakes

The combination of blueberries and corn is a big hit on a summer morning. Add grated orange zest for extra zing. The batter can be made ahead of time; leftover batter keeps well in an airtight container for up to two days. Serve the pancakes hot from the griddle with maple syrup and butter.

1 cup fresh or frozen sweet corn (leftover cooked or grilled corn is fine too)

3 large eggs

1½ cups milk

3 tablespoons melted butter

1 cup fresh or frozen blueberries

1 cup cornmeal

1 cup all-purpose flour

3 tablespoons sugar

1¼ teaspoons salt

1 teaspoon baking powder

If using fresh corn, bring 3 cups water to a boil in a medium pot. Add the corn kernels and blanch for 1 minute. Drain the corn and set aside.

In a bowl, whisk together the eggs, milk, and butter. Stir in the corn and blueberries. In another bowl, combine the cornmeal, flour, sugar, salt, and baking powder. Add the dry ingredients to the corn mixture and stir just until combined. Let stand for 15 minutes.

Heat a large nonstick skillet or griddle over medium-high heat. Grease lightly with canola oil. Working in batches, pour ½ cup of the batter for each pancake on the skillet. Cook for about 2 minutes, until the bottoms of pancakes are lightly browned. Flip and cook for about 2 minutes, or until pancakes are cooked through. Transfer to a warmed plate and repeat with the remaining batter, greasing the pan before each addition.

Serves 4

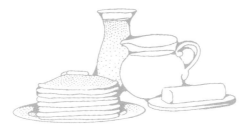

Blueberry Muffins

The course crystals of turbinado sugar give these delicate muffins an appealing crunch.

2 cups all-purpose flour
½ cup granulated sugar
2 teaspoons baking powder
1 teaspoon salt
1 egg, beaten
¼ cup unsalted butter, melted
1 cup milk
½ teaspoon pure vanilla extract
1¼ cups fresh blueberries
2 tablespoons turbinado sugar, for topping

Preheat the oven to 350°F. Lightly spray 12 muffin cups with vegetable-oil cooking spray or line with paper muffin cups. Combine the flour, granulated sugar, baking powder, and salt in a large bowl. In a separate bowl, mix the egg, butter, milk, and vanilla extract. Stir to combine well. Add the wet ingredients to the dry ingredients and stir just until combined. Do not overmix. Gently fold in the blueberries. Fill the muffin cups two-thirds full. Sprinkle each muffin with the turbinado sugar. Bake for 35 minutes, or until muffin tops are golden-brown and a toothpick inserted into the center of a muffin comes out clean. Cool for 5 minutes in the muffin tins, then unmold and transfer to a cooling rack. Serve warm. Freeze leftover muffins in plastic wrap or in a tightly sealed plastic bag for up to 2 months.

Makes 12 muffins

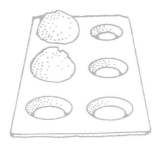

Blueberry Morning Glory Muffins

These muffins are packed with healthy ingredients. Make a batch and freeze them for days when the family needs breakfast on the run. Simply defrost for a minute in the microwave.

2 cups all-purpose flour

½ teaspoon salt

2 teaspoons baking soda

2 teaspoons ground cinnamon

¼ teaspoon ground cloves

⅛ teaspoon ground nutmeg

3 eggs, lightly beaten

1 cup canola oil

1¼ cups sugar

2 teaspoons pure vanilla extract

1 cup peeled and finely grated carrots

1 Granny Smith apple, peeled and grated

½ cup raisins

½ cup shredded coconut

¾ cup chopped pecans

1 cup fresh or thawed frozen blueberries

Preheat the oven to 350°F. Line 24 muffin tins with paper liners. In a small bowl, combine the flour, salt, baking soda, cinnamon, cloves, and nutmeg and mix well. In a large bowl, mix the eggs, oil, sugar, vanilla, carrots, apple, raisins, coconut, pecans, and blueberries. Add the dry ingredients and stir just until moistened.

Fill the muffin cups three-quarters of the way full and bake for 15 to 20 minutes, until a toothpick inserted into the center of a muffin comes out clean. Cool 5 minutes in tins, then transfer to cooling rack. Serve warm.

Makes 24 muffins

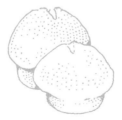

Salads, Sides, and Starters

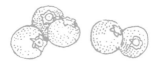

Blueberry–Blue Cheese Dip

This perfect blend of delicate sweetness and tangy, full-bodied flavor comes together in a snap, getting you out of the kitchen and on to having fun with family and friends. Serve with fresh raw vegetables, crackers, or apple slices.

6 ounces Danish blue or Maytag blue cheese, crumbled
1½ cups fresh or thawed frozen blueberries
8 ounces cream cheese
½ teaspoon salt
½ teaspoon freshly ground black pepper
¼ to ½ teaspoon hot chile sauce
½ cup finely sliced green onion, green part only
½ cup whole walnuts, chopped

Place the blue cheese and blueberries in the bowl of a food processor fitted with the metal blade and blend until smooth, about 2 minutes. Transfer the mixture to a bowl and stir in the remaining ingredients. To give the flavors time to meld, cover and refrigerate at least 1 hour or as long as 3 days.

Makes 3 cups

Spinach Salad with
Blueberry-Mustard Vinaigrette

With fresh berries added for extra color, this salad makes a wonderful accompaniment to grilled chicken or salmon.

Dressing

½ cup fresh blueberries

1 tablespoon sugar

2 tablespoons red wine vinegar

1 tablespoon peeled and minced red onion

½ tablespoon Dijon mustard

1 teaspoon freshly squeezed lemon juice

½ teaspoon salt

¼ teaspoon freshly ground black pepper

¼ cup olive oil

4 slices bacon

½ cup pecans

6 cups (5 ounces) baby spinach

½ cup peeled and thinly sliced red onion

½ cup crumbled blue cheese

To make the dressing, place the blueberries, sugar, vinegar, onion, mustard, lemon juice, salt, and pepper in the bowl of a food processor fitted with the metal blade. Process for 1 minute. Then, with the processor running, slowly add the oil in a steady stream, until the dressing is emulsified. Cover and place in the refrigerator until chilled, about 30 minutes. (The dressing will keep for up to 1 week in the refrigerator.)

Preheat a sauté pan over medium heat. Add the bacon slices. Cook, turning occasionally, until crispy, 12 to 15 minutes. Transfer strips to paper towels until cool enough to handle. Then place on cutting board and chop into crumbs with a knife.

To toast the pecans, preheat the oven to 400°F. Spread the pecans on a baking sheet in an even layer. Bake for 5 minutes, until golden and fragrant, paying very close attention to prevent burning. Transfer to cutting board and coarsely chop.

Combine the spinach, pecans, red onion, bacon, and blue cheese in a large bowl. Add 3 tablespoons of the dressing (reserve the remainder for another use). Toss to coat and serve immediately.

Serves 6

Pickled Onions, Avocado, Blueberries, and Sheep's Cheese Salad

Sheep's milk contains more than twice the fat of cow's milk (8½ percent compared to 4 percent), which is why it makes excellent, creamy cheese. Its richness balances the tartness of the blueberries and pickled onions.

½ red onion, peeled and thinly sliced

½ cup red wine vinegar

½ cup water

1 tablespoon sugar

⅛ teaspoon kosher salt

1 Hass avocado, peeled, pitted, and thinly sliced lengthwise

½ cup fresh blueberries

1 tablespoon extra virgin olive oil

Salt

4 ounces sheep's milk cheese, (Manchego, Idiazabal, or Pecorino) sliced into 8 pieces

Place the onion in a bowl. In a small saucepan, combine the vinegar, water, sugar, and salt over medium-high heat and bring to a boil. Pour the mixture over the onions and set aside for at least 1 hour. Then strain and discard juices.

When the onion has marinated, in a separate bowl, combine the avocado, blueberries, and onion. Drizzle the olive oil over the salad and add salt to taste. Divide among 4 plates. Place 2 slices of the cheese on top of each salad. Serve immediately.

Serves 4

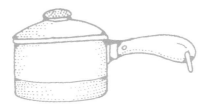

Arugula, Prosciutto, and Blueberry Salad with Honey-Citrus Vinaigrette

The sweetness of the blueberries and the honey dressing complements the peppery flavor of arugula, while the salty prosciutto adds an interesting kick. For a slight variation, add chopped beets or melon.

Dressing

1 tablespoon minced shallots

1 teaspoon honey

1 tablespoon freshly squeezed orange juice

¼ cup extra virgin olive oil

¼ teaspoon finely chopped fresh mint

1 teaspoon finely chopped fresh thyme

½ teaspoon salt

2½ ounces arugula

½ cup fresh blueberries

8 thin slices prosciutto, cut into ¼-inch strips

Place all of the ingredients for the dressing in a bowl and combine well with a whisk.

In a separate large bowl, place the arugula, blueberries, and prosciutto. Add 3 tablespoons of the dressing and toss well (reserve the remainder for another use). Divide among 4 plates and serve immediately.

Serves 4

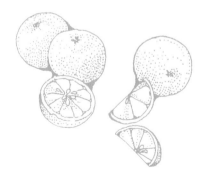

Mesclun Greens with Toasted Almonds and Blueberry-Basil Vinaigrette

Mesclun is another word for mixed. *This salad is most delicious when the mesclun is a balanced mix of sweet, peppery, and grassy greens. Mesclun greens are best kept refrigerated in an airtight container or sealed plastic bag layered with paper towels.*

1 cup sliced almonds
½ cup fresh blueberries
2 tablespoons water
1 tablespoon red wine vinegar
½ teaspoon kosher salt
1 tablespoon minced shallot
¼ cup extra virgin olive oil
1 tablespoon basil chiffonade
10 cups loosely packed mesclun greens

To toast the almonds, preheat the oven to 400°F. Spread the almonds on a baking sheet in an even layer. Bake in the oven for 5 minutes, or until golden and fragrant, watching closely to avoid burning.

To make the dressing, combine the blueberries, water, vinegar, and salt in the bowl of a food processor fitted with the metal blade. Blend, scraping the sides of the processor as necessary, for 1 minute, or until the blueberries are puréed. Add the shallot, oil, and basil. Pulse until well combined.

Place the greens and almonds in a large bowl. Add 5 to 6 tablespoons of the dressing and toss well. (Reserve the remainder for another use. Store dressing in refrigerator for up to 30 days.) Divide the salad among 4 plates and serve.

Serves 4

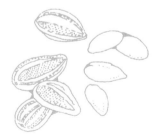

Goat Cheese Tart with Caramelized Onions and Blueberries

Perfect for a light lunch, this tart goes well with a green salad or as part of a larger buffet. Make the tarts a day ahead, cover in plastic wrap, and store in the fridge. Always bring them to room temperature before serving.

Crust

⅓ cup walnuts

1 cup all-purpose flour

1 teaspoon sugar

¼ teaspoon salt

¼ teaspoon dried thyme

⅛ teaspoon freshly ground black pepper

¼ teaspoon baking powder

6 tablespoons cold unsalted butter, cut into small pieces

1 egg

1 tablespoon freshly squeezed lemon juice

Filling

3 tablespoons canola oil

3 yellow onions, peeled and thinly sliced

5 ounces soft goat cheese

6 ounces cream cheese

¼ teaspoon dried thyme

⅛ teaspoon freshly ground black pepper

½ teaspoon salt

2 eggs

½ cup heavy whipping cream

1¼ cups fresh or thawed frozen blueberries

2 tablespoons chopped fresh chives

To make the crust, roast the walnuts in a sauté pan over medium-low heat. Stir often until they begin to color and become aromatic. Remove from the pan and set aside to cool. Place the flour, sugar, salt, thyme, pepper, baking powder, and roasted walnuts in the bowl of a food processor fitted with the metal blade and pulse to combine. Add the butter and pulse until the mixture resembles course crumbs. Place the egg and lemon juice in a small bowl and whisk to combine. Add to the flour mixture in a steady stream while pulsing. Pulse until just combined and a ball of dough forms.

Coat a 10-inch tart pan with vegetable-oil cooking spray. Sprinkle the dough lightly with flour. With floured

(continued)

hands, press the dough into the pan. Refrigerate the crust for 45 to 60 minutes.

Preheat the oven to 375°F. Prick the crust all over with a fork. Bake for about 15 minutes, or until lightly browned. Remove from the oven and decrease the oven temperature to 325°F. Allow the crust to cool.

To make the filling, heat the oil in a heavy saucepan over medium-high heat. Add the onions and cook, stirring frequently, for 20 to 30 minutes, until they are deep brown and reduced in volume by at least two-thirds. Transfer to a bowl and allow to cool.

Place the onions, goat cheese, cream cheese, thyme, pepper, and salt in the bowl of the food processor fitted with the metal blade and pulse to combine. When smooth, add the eggs and heavy cream, and pulse just to mix well.

Place the berries evenly over the crust and cover with the filling mixture. Sprinkle the chives over the top. Place in the oven and bake for 25 to 30 minutes, until the surface is slightly brown and the filling is completely set. Remove from the oven and allow to cool on a cooling rack. Serve warm or at room temperature.

Serves 10 to 12

Entrées

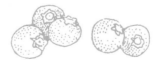

Pork Tenderloin with Peach-Blueberry Chutney

Make the chutney ahead of time so its many ingredients have time to meld together. Sparkling cider is an excellent pairing with this dish.

Chutney

1 cup fresh or frozen blueberries

1 large peach, with skin, pitted and chopped

1 cup peeled and finely chopped yellow onion

½ cup red wine vinegar

¼ cup golden raisins

¼ cup packed dark brown sugar

2 teaspoons yellow mustard seed

1 teaspoon minced fresh ginger

½ teaspoon ground cinnamon

⅛ teaspoon salt

⅛ teaspoon ground nutmeg

2 (1- to 1¼-pound) pork tenderloins

1 tablespoon minced lemon zest

Salt and freshly ground black pepper

To make the chutney, in a saucepan, combine the blueberries, peach, onion, vinegar, raisins, sugar, mustard seed, ginger, cinnamon, salt, and nutmeg. Bring to a boil over medium-high heat. Decrease the heat to medium and simmer, stirring occasionally, for about 1 hour, or until thickened. Remove from the heat and keep warm. (Or refrigerate the chutney for up to 30 days.)

To grill the meat, prepare a fire in a charcoal grill or preheat a gas grill to medium-high. (If using an oven, preheat to 400°F.) Rub the tenderloins with the lemon zest, brush with canola oil, and generously sprinkle with salt and pepper. Place on the grill rack and cook, turning once, for 6 to 8 minutes on each side, or until just cooked through. (If using an oven, coat a large ovenproof skillet with 2 to 3 tablespoons canola oil and heat on medium-high. Add the meat and sear on all sides. Cook for 1 to 2 minutes, until meat is dark brown. Transfer to the oven and roast for 10 minutes.) Let the meat rest for 5 minutes before slicing. Serve the pork with chutney on the side.

Serves 4 to 6

Herbed Tuna Salad with Berries

Rich in health-promoting antioxidants and vitamins, this salad is a bright take on tuna. So cool and refreshing, it is the perfect summer entrée.

2 (16-ounce) cans white or light tuna, packed in water

1 celery stalk, thinly sliced

¼ cup peeled and minced red onion

2½ tablespoons finely chopped fresh dill

½ cup chopped cucumber

⅓ cup finely chopped red bell pepper

½ cup fresh blueberries

8 large leaves lettuce, for serving

Dressing

3 tablespoons mayonnaise

1½ tablespoons red wine vinegar

½ tablespoon freshly squeezed lemon juice

½ teaspoon Dijon mustard

¼ teaspoon salt

¼ teaspoon freshly ground black pepper

Place the tuna, celery, onion, dill, cucumber, and bell pepper in a bowl and toss well to combine. In a small bowl, combine the dressing ingredients with a whisk. Pour the dressing over the tuna mixture and toss to coat. Cover and place in the refrigerator until chilled. Just before serving, add the blueberries and toss gently. Serve on a bed of lettuce.

Serves 4

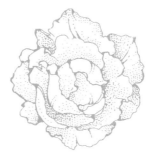

Grilled Swordfish with Blueberry-Verbena Butter

For a change, use red snapper or salmon in place of swordfish. The best lemon verbena comes freshly picked from the garden.

¼ cup unsalted butter, at room temperature
½ cup fresh or partially thawed frozen blueberries
⅛ teaspoon kosher salt
¼ cup young lemon verbena leaves, finely chopped
1 tablespoon minced shallot
4 (6-ounce, 1-inch-thick) swordfish steaks
2 tablespoons vegetable oil
Salt and freshly ground black pepper

With the back of a fork or in the bowl of a food processor fitted with the metal blade, blend the butter, blueberries, and salt until completely blended. This may take up to 2 minutes in the food processor. Transfer the butter mixture to a bowl. Fold in the verbena and shallot. Cover and refrigerate for at least 1 hour to allow the flavors to develop. (Store the butter in the refrigerator for up to 1 month or freeze it for up to 3 months.)

Prepare a fire in a charcoal grill or preheat a gas grill to medium-high. Rub the fish with the oil and season with salt and pepper to taste. Place the fish on the grill rack and cook, turning once, for about 5 minutes on each side. The swordfish is ready when it has turned from translucent to opaque throughout. Transfer the fish to plates. Place 1 tablespoon of the blueberry verbena butter on each steak. Serve immediately.

Serves 4

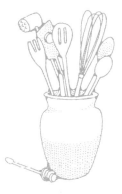

New York Strip Steak with Blueberry-Port Sauce

This rich blueberry sauce also tastes wonderful over duck, chicken, or lamb. Thyme and mint are excellent substitutions for the rosemary.

2 tablespoons minced shallots
1 cup fresh or thawed frozen blueberries
1½ cups port
1 cup beef broth
2 teaspoons sugar
1 teaspoon chopped fresh rosemary
1 tablespoon unsalted butter
4 (8-ounce) New York strip steaks
2 tablespoons canola oil
Salt and freshly ground black pepper

In a saucepan, combine the shallots, blueberries, port, broth, and sugar, and bring to a boil over medium-high heat. Boil for about 1 hour, until reduced to ½ cup. Remove from the heat and stir in the rosemary and butter. Keep warm.

Prepare a fire in a charcoal grill or preheat a grill to high. Pat the steaks dry, brush both sides with the oil, and season to taste with salt and pepper. Place on the grill rack and cook for 4 to 5 minutes on each side for medium-rare. Remove from the heat and set aside to rest for 5 minutes. Place 1 steak on each place and drizzle 2 tablespoons of the sauce over each. Serve immediately.

Serves 4

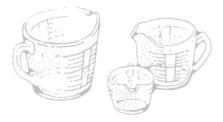

Roasted Chicken Salad with Walnuts, Apples, and Dried Blueberries

This salad is more delicious made twenty-four hours ahead of time so the flavors have time to develop and deepen. Roasting the chicken with the skin on and bone in results in flavorful, juicy meat. Add it to the salad when the meat is still slightly warm, as warm chicken absorbs the dressing and picks up flavors better than cold chicken.

Mayonnaise

1 egg

1 tablespoon cider vinegar

¼ teaspoon salt

¼ teaspoon Dijon mustard

1 cup canola oil

Salad

2 (1-pound) chicken breasts, with skin

½ teaspoon kosher salt, plus more as needed

Freshly ground black pepper

1 celery stalk, diced

½ cup walnuts

½ cup dried blueberries

½ cup diced red apple (such as a Braeburn, Gravenstein, Macoun, Empire), with peel

¼ cup finely chopped fresh parsley

2 scallions, white and light green parts, finely chopped

¼ cup plain whole milk yogurt

1 cup chopped Romaine lettuce, for serving

To make the mayonnaise, place the egg, vinegar, salt, and mustard in the bowl of a food processor fitted with a metal blade. Blend on medium speed until well mixed. Add the oil in a slow but steady stream until emulsified. Set aside.

For the salad, preheat the oven to 400°F. Season the chicken breasts on both sides with salt and pepper. Place them on a sheet pan with no oil. Roast in the oven for 30 minutes, turning them over halfway through. Remove from oven and set aside for 10 minutes.

While the chicken is cooking, assemble the salad. Combine the ½ teaspoon salt with ¼ cup of the mayonnaise, the celery, walnuts, blueberries, apple, parsley, scallions, and yogurt in a large bowl and mix well to combine. Cover with plastic wrap and place in the refrigerator.

(continued)

Remove the skin from the chicken and chop the meat into bite-size chunks or shred into bite-size pieces. Add to the salad and toss, making sure the chicken is well coated with the dressing. Serve as is, or cover and refrigerate until ready to serve. Divide into portions on a bed of Romaine.

Serves 4

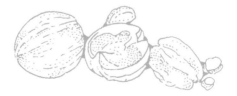

Grilled Venison with Ancho Chile–Blueberry Sauce

Venison is similar to beef but much leaner, a great alternative for those looking for a healthier choice. The combination of blueberries and venison dates back to the Native Americans in the Northwest Territories. Legend has it, one of Lewis and Clark's first meals with the natives of the Northwest was venison cured with blueberries.

Ancho Purée

2 ancho chiles

2 cups water

½ teaspoon salt

2 tablespoons unsalted butter

1 celery stalk, finely chopped

1 carrot, peeled and finely chopped

½ cup peeled and finely chopped yellow onion

½ teaspoon salt

½ cup port

2 tablespoons light brown sugar

(continued)

2 cups chicken broth

1 cup fresh blueberries

4 (4-ounce) venison medallions

2 tablespoons vegetable oil

1½ teaspoons kosher salt, plus extra

Freshly ground black pepper

To make the purée, place the chiles in a small bowl. In a small saucepan, bring the water to a boil over high heat. Pour over the chiles and let steep for 1 hour. Remove the chiles, reserving ¼ cup of the soaking liquid. Stem and seed the chiles and place in the bowl of a food processor fitted with the metal blade. Add the salt and the soaking liquid. Process for about 1 minute, or until smooth, scraping down the sides as needed. (If desired, make the purée ahead and refrigerate for up to 30 days.)

To make the sauce, melt 1 tablespoon of the butter in a saucepan over medium heat. Add the celery, carrot, onion, and salt, and sauté for 3 to 5 minutes, until soft. Add the ancho purée, port, brown sugar, and broth. Increase the heat to medium-high and cook, stirring occasionally, for about 20 minutes, or until reduced to 1 cup. Pass through a fine-mesh sieve into a clean saucepan, add the blue-berries, and cook over medium heat for 12 minutes. Add the remaining 1 tablespoon butter and stir until combined. Season to taste with salt and pepper. Keep warm.

Prepare a fire in a charcoal grill or preheat a gas grill to medium-high. Pat the venison medallions dry with paper towels. Place the meat on a plate and coat both sides with the oil. Sprinkle both sides with the 1½ teaspoon salt. Place on the grill rack and grill for 2 to 3 minutes on each side, until just cooked to medium-rare. Slice each medallion on an angle into 4 to 6 pieces. Divide among 4 plates. Drizzle 1 to 2 tablespoons of the sauce over the top. Serve immediately.

Serves 4

Spreads, Sauces, Jams, and Gifts

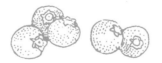

Blueberry Salsa

Serve this spicy fruit salsa with grilled fish or chicken. Add a dash of hot sauce to kick it up a notch.

1 cup fresh or frozen blueberries, coarsely chopped
½ red bell pepper, seeded, deribbed, and diced
1 jalapeño or serrano chile, minced
2 tablespoons minced cilantro
2 green onions, white and light green parts, finely chopped
Juice of ½ lime
¼ teaspoon kosher salt
Pinch of sugar

Combine all of the ingredients in a medium bowl and toss well. Refrigerate for 30 minutes before serving. Cover and refrigerate for up to 3 days.

Makes about 1 cup

Blueberry Jam

This jam tastes like it took hours to make, but it goes from pan to jar in under 30 minutes. Double the recipe so you can save some for dark winter mornings, a reminder that summer will be back.

2 cups fresh or thawed frozen blueberries
1 tablespoon pectin
1 tablespoon honey
1 tablespoon freshly squeezed lemon juice
½ cup water
1 cup sugar

Combine all of the ingredients in a saucepan and bring to a boil over medium-high heat. Continue to boil, stirring occasionally, for 12 minutes, or until the mixture begins to gel. To test the consistency, chill a small plate in the freezer for 15 minutes. Remove the plate from the freezer and drop small amounts of the jam onto it. The jam is ready when it holds its shape instead of pooling out over the plate. Transfer to clean jars with tightly fitting lids and refrigerate for 30 days.

Note: Sterilizing and sealing the jars keeps jam fresh for up to a year. Those who plan to keep the jam for an extended period should sterilize a jar and its lid by using a pair of tongs to submerge them in boiling water for at least 10 minutes. Alternatively, place the jar, lid, and metal soup spoon in the oven at 250°F for 25 minutes. Remove from the oven and, wearing oven mitts, use the sterile spoon to scoop the jam from the pan and into the jars. Still using mitts, tightly screw on the lid, and set aside to cool. The hot air between the jam and the lid contracts as it cools, sealing the lid tight. The jam is now safely stored at room temperature. Once the jar is opened, place the jam in the refrigerator and use within 30 days.

Makes about 1½ cups

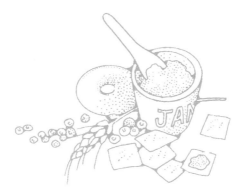

Blueberry Granola

Homemade granola is delicious and extremely easy to make. Try it sprinkled on yogurt and fruit salad or ice cream, or enjoy it as a hearty breakfast cereal.

⅔ cup canola oil
⅔ cup honey
¼ cup packed light brown sugar
6 cups old-fashioned oats
1 teaspoon ground cinnamon
1 cup unsalted raw shelled sunflower seeds
2 tablespoons sesame seeds
½ cup sliced almonds
1 cup dried blueberries

Position the oven racks to divide the oven evenly in thirds and preheat the oven to 350°F. Have 2 ungreased baking sheets ready.

Place the oil, honey, and sugar in a bowl and whisk to combine. Place the oats, cinnamon, sunflower seeds, and sesame seeds in a large bowl and stir to mix. Pour the honey mixture into the oats mixture and toss well to combine and coat. Divide evenly between the baking sheets and spread in an even layer.

Bake for 30 minutes, varying the pans' positions and stirring every 10 minutes to allow for even baking, until the granola is golden and toasted. Remove from the oven, stir to loosen, and let cool on the pans, stirring occasionally to keep the granola from sticking. When completely cool, transfer to a large bowl and add the almonds and blueberries. Store in an airtight container for up to 2 weeks.

Makes about 8 cups

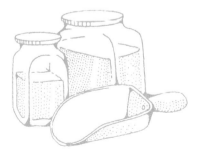

Savory Blueberry Breadsticks

A fine alternative to crackers, these flavorful breadsticks are a festive and colorful addition to any menu. Serve them with soup or salad, and watch them disappear! Kids like to help with this recipe—small hands are great at rolling dough.

2 tablespoons olive oil

⅓ cup peeled and finely chopped red onion

1 tablespoon minced garlic

3½ cups all-purpose flour, plus more for kneading

1½ teaspoons kosher salt, plus more for sprinkling

½ teaspoon freshly ground black pepper

1 cup fresh or frozen blueberries

2 teaspoons active dry yeast

¼ teaspoon sugar

¾ cup hot water (120° to 130°F)

In a skillet, heat the oil over medium heat. Add the onion and garlic and sauté for about 10 minutes, or until the onion is soft. Remove from the heat and let cool.

Mix together the flour, 1½ teaspoons salt, and pepper in a small bowl and set aside. Place the blueberries in the bowl of a food processor fitted with the metal blade and purée until smooth. Set aside.

In a large bowl, mix together the yeast and sugar. Stir in the hot water, continuing to stir just until the yeast dissolves. Let rest until the yeast mixture becomes foamy, about 10 minutes. Gently stir the onion mixture and the blueberry purée into the yeast. Add the flour mixture and stir to combine just until a dough ball forms.

Lightly grease a large bowl with canola oil. Working on a lightly floured surface with lightly floured hands, knead the dough until elastic, about 5 minutes. Place the dough ball in the oiled bowl and turn to coat. Place a damp kitchen towel over the dough and place the bowl in a warm place to rise for 45 minutes, or until approximately doubled in volume.

Preheat the oven to 350°F. Remove the dough from the bowl and roll it into a rectangle about ½ inch thick and 15 inches long, then cut into 24 to 30 pieces. Working on a lightly floured surface, roll the pieces of dough into 15-inch-long ropes, about the thickness of your pinky finger. Arrange breadsticks on baking sheets 2 inches apart

(continued)

and brush their tops with water and sprinkle with kosher salt. Bake for 45 to 55 minutes, until very crispy and slightly browned. Serve warm. The breadsticks stay fresh in an airtight container for up to 2 weeks.

Makes 24 to 30 breadsticks

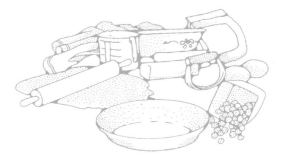

Blueberry-Mint Vinegar

Use this vinegar in a dressing for an arugula or spinach salad, or as a marinade, glaze, or reduction for pork, ham, or duck. The beautiful plum color makes it an ideal gift item. Add fresh blueberries for decorative purposes.

1 tablespoon honey
1 cup white wine vinegar
½ cup fresh mint leaves
1 cup fresh or thawed frozen blueberries

Combine the honey and vinegar in a small, nonreactive saucepan and bring to a boil over high heat. Place the mint and blueberries in a glass bowl and pour the honey and vinegar mixture over them. Cover and let sit at room temperature for 2 days. Pass through a fine-mesh strainer and discard the solids. Cover tightly and store in the refrigerator. The vinegar is best when used within 30 days.

Makes 1 cup

Desserts

Coconut-Blueberry Ice Cream

This richly flavored ice cream pairs the tartness of blueberries with the smooth, soothing flavor of coconut. It's a dessert no one will forget.

½ cup milk

½ cup heavy whipping cream

1 cup coconut milk

½ cup granulated sugar

1 cup fresh or partially thawed frozen blueberries

4 egg yolks

In a medium saucepan, bring the milk, heavy cream, coconut milk, and ¼ cup of the sugar to a simmer over medium-high heat. Simmer for 3 minutes. Remove from the heat and add the blueberries, mashing them lightly with the back of a fork. Let cool to room temperature, at least 3 hours. Strain out the blueberries. With a handheld electric mixer, whip the egg yolks and the remaining ¼ cup of the sugar on high speed for 3 minutes. Add to the coconut mixture and refrigerate for at least 3 hours and for up to 24 hours. Freeze in an ice cream maker according to the manufacturer's instructions.

Makes 1 pint

Lemon-Blueberry Pound Cake

This pound cake doubles as breakfast and dessert. For dessert, serve it with heavy cream drizzled on top or with freshly whipped cream.

1¼ cups all-purpose flour

1 teaspoon baking powder

¼ teaspoon salt

½ cup unsalted butter, at room temperature

¾ cup sugar

2 eggs

¼ cup heavy whipping cream

¼ cup freshly squeezed lemon juice

1 cup fresh or frozen blueberries

Preheat the oven to 350°F. Coat a 4 by 8-inch loaf pan with vegetable oil cooking spray.

Place the flour, baking powder, and salt in a bowl and mix well. In the bowl of an electric mixer fitted with a whisk attachment, or using a whisk to stir by hand, cream the butter with the sugar. Add 1 egg at a time, beating to fully incorporate each. Add half of the flour mixture, then add the heavy cream and lemon juice. Mix just until smooth. Add the remaining flour mixture and stir until just combined. Using a wooden spoon, gently fold in the blueberries. Pour the batter into the prepared pan and bake for 1 hour and 20 minutes. The cake is done when a toothpick inserted in the center comes out clean.

Remove the cake from the oven and let cool in the pan for 10 minutes. Transfer to cooling rack for 5 minutes and serve. If desired, store the cake in the refrigerator for 3 days or wrap in aluminum foil or plastic wrap and freeze for up to 2 months.

Makes one 4 by 8-inch loaf

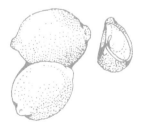

Melon and Blueberry Salad with White Wine, Vanilla, and Mint

This summer dessert is light and refreshing, with a touch of sophistication. Serve with sugar cookies, pound cake, or shortbread.

1½ cups dry white wine

½ cup sugar

1 vanilla bean, split in half lengthwise

½ cantaloupe, seeded, peeled, and cut in large dice (about 2⅓ cups)

½ honeydew, seeded, peeled, and cut in large dice (about 2⅓ cups)

½ watermelon, seeded, peeled, and cut in large dice (about 2⅓ cups)

1 mango, pitted, peeled, and cut in large dice

2 cups fresh blueberries

½ cup chopped fresh mint, plus additional sprigs for garnish

Combine ½ cup of the wine with the sugar in a small saucepan. Scrape in the seeds from the vanilla bean and add the bean. Cook over low heat, stirring continuously, until the sugar dissolves and the syrup is hot, about 2 minutes. Transfer from the heat and let steep in the pan for 30 minutes. Remove the vanilla bean from the syrup and discard.

Combine all of the fruit and the chopped mint in a large bowl. Add the vanilla syrup to the remaining 1 cup wine, stir to combine, and pour over the fruit. Toss lightly. Cover and refrigerate for at least 3 hours.

To serve, spoon some of the chilled fruit and liquid into 6 goblets or spoon over pound cake. Garnish with a mint sprig and serve immediately.

Serves 6

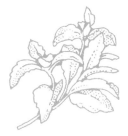

Blueberry-Vanilla Biscotti

Blueberry and vanilla go together as well as coffee and cream. However, for something different and just as delicious, substitute maple or lemon extract for the vanilla.

2 cups all-purpose flour, plus ½ cup
  for working the dough
2 teaspoons baking powder
¼ teaspoon salt
¼ teaspoon ground cinnamon
1 cup dried blueberries
3 large eggs
1 cup sugar
2 teaspoons pure vanilla extract

Preheat the oven to 350°F. Place the flour, baking powder, salt, and cinnamon in a large bowl and stir with a spoon to mix well. Add the blueberries and stir to mix. In another large bowl, whisk together the eggs, sugar, and vanilla extract until smooth. Gradually add the dry ingredients to the wet ingredients and stir to mix well.

Line a baking sheet with parchment paper. Lightly dust a work surface with flour. Place the dough on the work surface and sprinkle lightly with more of the flour to prevent your hands from sticking to the dough. Knead the dough 4 or 5 times and, using your hands, shape into a log about 12 inches long and 4 inches wide. Place the dough on the prepared baking sheet and bake for 40 minutes, until firm to the touch.

Remove the baked loaf from the oven and keep the oven on. Cool the loaf on a wire rack. With a large metal spatula, transfer the loaf to a wire rack to cool.

Line a baking sheet with parchment paper. When the loaf is cool, using a serrated knife, slice into ¼-inch slices. Place the slices on the prepared baking sheet and bake for 10 to 15 minutes. Turn the biscotti and bake for another 10 to 15 minutes, until crispy.

Keep extra biscotti in an airtight container for up to 30 days or freeze for up to 2 months.

Makes 18 biscotti

Blueberry Buckle

Serve this versatile cake with coffee at brunch or for a snack in the afternoon. In the evening, it makes an irresistible dessert warmed and with a scoop of vanilla ice cream.

Topping

1 cup packed light brown sugar

⅔ cup all-purpose flour

1½ teaspoons ground cinnamon

6 tablespoons salted butter, cold, cut into small pieces

Cake

2 cups all-purpose flour

2 teaspoons baking powder

½ teaspoon salt

½ cup salted butter, at room temperature

½ cup sugar

1 egg

1½ teaspoons pure vanilla extract

½ cup milk

2 cups fresh or partially thawed frozen blueberries

To make the topping, combine the brown sugar, flour, and cinnamon in a small bowl. Using a pastry blender or your fingers, cut in the cold butter until the mixture is crumbly. Set aside.

To make the cake, preheat the oven to 350°F. Butter and flour a 9-inch springform pan. Place the flour, baking powder, and salt in a small bowl and stir to mix. Place the butter in a large bowl and beat with a spoon until creamy. Add the sugar and beat until fluffy. Beat in the egg and vanilla. Add the flour mixture alternately with the milk, beating well after each addition. With a spoon, gently fold in the berries until well distributed.

Spread the batter into the prepared pan and cover evenly with the topping. Bake for 55 to 60 minutes, until the topping is a deep golden brown. The cake is done when a toothpick inserted into the center comes out clean.

Remove from the oven and place the cake on a wire rack to cool in the pan. To remove the cake, run a knife around the edge of the pan and remove the bottom. Serve warm or cover with plastic wrap and refrigerate. Bring to room temperature after refrigerating, or warm in the oven at 350°F for 10 minutes.

Serves 8 to 12

Lemon–Poppy Seed Cake with Blueberry Compote

Bakers have added poppy seeds to cakes for hundreds of years...and for good reason. The seeds provide just the right amount of delicate texture and nutty flavor. While the cake alone is moist, it's made more luscious with the addition of fruit.

Blueberry Compote

½ cup water

½ cup sugar

2 tablespoons freshly squeezed lemon juice

1 teaspoon pure vanilla extract

2½ cups fresh or thawed frozen blueberries

1 cup strawberries, hulled and quartered

2 large nectarines, pitted and cut into wedges

Cake

1¼ cups all-purpose flour

⅔ cup sugar

½ cup cornstarch

1½ tablespoons poppy seeds

2½ teaspoons baking powder

1 teaspoon salt
2 tablespoons butter
1 large egg
1 cup skim milk
2 teaspoons freshly grated lemon zest
1 teaspoon pure vanilla extract

To make the compote, place the water, sugar, and lemon juice in a small saucepan and bring to a boil over medium heat. Continue to boil, stirring occasionally, until the sugar is dissolved, about 2 minutes. Remove from the heat and cool until just slightly warm. Stir in the vanilla, blueberries, strawberries, and nectarines. Transfer to a small bowl and refrigerate.

To make the cake, preheat the oven to 350°F. Grease an 8-inch cake pan with butter and dust with flour. In a large bowl, combine the flour, sugar, cornstarch, poppy seeds, baking powder, and salt. Using a pastry blender or your fingers, blend in the butter until incorporated. In a small bowl, beat the egg lightly with a whisk, and stir in the milk, lemon zest, and vanilla. Stir the milk mixture into the flour mixture just until blended, then pour into

(continued)

the pan. Bake for 35 minutes, or until a toothpick inserted into the center of the cake comes out clean.

Remove the cake from the oven and let cool in the pan for 10 minutes. Run a knife around the edge and bottom of the pan to loosen the cake, and transfer to a wire rack to cool.

Serve the cake on individual plates topped with ½ cup of the chilled fruit compote.

Serves 8

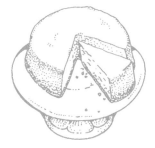

Blueberry Cream Cheese Tart

A tasty alternative to cheesecake, these small individual tarts are easy to make and beautiful to serve. Or, if preferred, make this recipe into one large tart.

Crust

½ cup unsalted butter

½ cup confectioners' sugar

1 teaspoon pure vanilla extract

1¼ cups all-purpose flour

1 teaspoon salt

⅛ teaspoon ground cinnamon

Filling

¾ cup heavy whipping cream

½ cup granulated sugar

4 egg yolks

1½ tablespoons cornstarch

¼ cup milk

8 ounces cream cheese

1 teaspoon pure vanilla extract

2½ cups fresh or thawed frozen blueberries

(continued)

To make the crust, in the bowl of an electric mixer fitted with the paddle attachment, beat the butter, confectioners' sugar, and vanilla on medium-high speed until creamy and smooth, about 3 minutes. Add the flour, salt, and cinnamon until just combined. Turn the dough out onto a lightly floured surface and gather into a ball. Flatten into a disk, cover with plastic wrap, and refrigerate for 3 hours.

Preheat the oven to 300°F. Divide the dough into 4 equal pieces. Using your hands, press the dough into 4-inch tart pans, to $\frac{1}{8}$ inch thick. Prick the dough all over with a fork and bake for 15 minutes, until golden brown. Remove from the oven and set aside to cool.

To make the filling, combine the cream and 6 tablespoons of the sugar in a saucepan. Bring to a simmer over medium heat. In a separate bowl, whisk together the egg yolks, cornstarch, and milk. Add a little of the hot cream mixture to the egg yolk mixture to warm it, whisking constantly. Pour the egg mixture into the cream mixture, whisking constantly. Return to the stove over medium-high heat and bring to a boil, continuing to whisk. Cook for 2 minutes, until the mixture thickens. Add the cream cheese and vanilla and whisk until smooth. Cover with plastic wrap and refrigerate until chilled and set.

Place 1 cup of the blueberries and the remaining 2 tablespoons sugar in a saucepan. Cook over medium heat until the berries are broken down, about 5 minutes. Strain out the blueberries, leaving blueberry syrup. Add the remaining 1½ cups blueberries to the berry syrup and toss to combine.

Divide the cream cheese filling evenly among the 4 tart shells. Divide the blueberries over the top of the cheese filling and serve immediately.

Serves 4

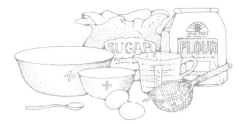

Steamed Blueberry Pudding

Don't wait for a special occasion to make this elegant dessert. For an alcohol-free alternative to the sauce, serve the pudding with French vanilla lowfat frozen yogurt or ice cream.

Sauce

½ cup salted butter

1½ cups confectioners' sugar, sifted

2 tablespoons brandy

Cake

1½ cups all-purpose flour

½ teaspoon salt

½ teaspoon baking powder

½ teaspoon baking soda

⅛ teaspoon ground cloves

¼ teaspoon ground nutmeg

½ teaspoon ground cinnamon

⅓ cup molasses

¼ cup sugar

2 tablespoons brandy

2 tablespoons vegetable oil

1 cup fresh or thawed frozen blueberries

1 Granny Smith apple, coarsely peeled

¼ cup currants

To make the sauce, melt the butter in a small saucepan, remove from heat, and add the sugar and brandy. Whisk until smooth. Set aside. When the pudding is ready, reheat the sauce over medium-low heat to prevent scalding.

To make the pudding, thoroughly butter a 6-cup pudding mold. In a large bowl, add the flour, salt, baking powder, baking soda, cloves, nutmeg, and cinnamon and mix well. Place the molasses, sugar, brandy, and oil in a separate bowl and mix well to combine. Stir in the blueberries, apple, and currants. Add the fruit mixture to the flour mixture and stir just until blended. Spoon into the mold. Cover the mold tightly with aluminum foil and place on a rack in a Dutch oven or steamer. Pour in enough boiling water to reach halfway up the mold. Cover the Dutch oven and set over medium heat. Cook, keeping the water at a simmer, for about 2 hours, or until a wooden toothpick inserted in the center comes out clean. Remove the pudding mold from the Dutch oven and let stand for

(continued)

5 minutes. Invert the mold onto a serving plate. If it does not come out right away, leave the mold inverted and allow to fall out on its own. Serve the pudding warm with the brandy sauce drizzled on top.

Note: If desired, make the pudding several days ahead and refrigerate for up to 1 week or freeze for 30 days. To freeze, cover in plastic wrap, then cover in aluminum foil. Thaw the frozen pudding before reheating. To reheat, remove the foil and plastic, and rewrap in foil. Heat in a preheated 350°F oven for 30 to 45 minutes. Serve topped with the warmed sauce.

Serves 8 to 12

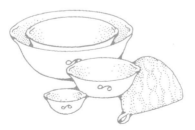

Blueberry-Lemon Tart with Whipped Cream

Blueberries and lemon are a marriage made in heaven. This tart has a rich layer of blueberry-studded lemon custard. Finish it with a dollop of sweet whipped cream.

Crust

1⅔ cups all-purpose flour

2 tablespoons sugar

2 teaspoons grated lemon zest

⅛ teaspoon salt

½ cup unsalted butter, cold, cut into ½-inch pieces

3 to 4 tablespoons cold water

Filling

3 large eggs

½ cup sugar

1½ teaspoons cornstarch

⅓ cup heavy whipping cream

⅓ cup freshly squeezed lemon juice

Salt

2 cups fresh or thawed frozen blueberries

(continued)

Whipped Cream

½ cup heavy whipping cream

1 teaspoon sugar

½ teaspoon pure vanilla extract

To make the crust, place the flour, sugar, lemon zest, and salt in the bowl of a food processor fitted with the metal blade and process to combine. Add the butter through the feeder tube, cutting it in with pulses until the mixture resembles coarse crumbs. Mix in enough cold water to form a dough, adding 1 tablespoon at a time and mixing. Turn the dough out onto a lightly floured surface and gather into a ball. Flatten into a disk, cover in plastic wrap, and refrigerate for 45 minutes.

Preheat the oven to 400°F. Roll the dough out on a lightly floured surface to form a 15-inch circle. Transfer the dough to an 11-inch tart pan that has a removable bottom. Press the dough into place. Trim the dough to overhang ½ inch. Fold the overhang back on itself to form a double layer on the sides. Place in the freezer for 15 minutes.

Preheat the oven to 400°F. Remove the crust from the freezer and bake for 16 to 18 minutes, until pale golden brown. Transfer to wire cooling rack and let cool. Keep the oven on.

To make the filling, whisk the eggs, sugar, cornstarch, heavy cream, lemon juice, and salt in a bowl to blend well. Gently stir in the blueberries. Pour the filling into the crust, making sure to evenly distribute the berries on the crust. Return the pan to the oven and bake for 20 to 23 minutes, until set. Remove from the oven and cool completely on a wire rack.

To make the whipped cream, combine the heavy cream, sugar, and vanilla in a small bowl. Using a hand-held mixer, whip until soft peaks form. Serve the tart at room temperature topped with the whipped cream.

Serves 8 to 10

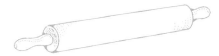

Blueberry Layer Cake with Cream Cheese Frosting

Beautiful and moist, this decadent creation makes a great summer birthday cake. If desired, make it a day ahead, cover with a cake dome, and store in the refrigerator.

Cake

3 cups all-purpose flour

⅓ cup cornstarch

¾ teaspoon baking powder

½ teaspoon baking soda

½ teaspoon salt

¾ cup unsalted butter, at room temperature

2 cups sugar

4 large eggs, at room temperature

¼ cup freshly squeezed lemon juice

1½ teaspoons packed grated lemon zest

1 teaspoon pure vanilla extract

¼ cup plus 2 tablespoons buttermilk

2½ cups fresh or partially thawed frozen blueberries

Frosting

12 ounces cream cheese, at room temperature

½ cup unsalted butter, at room temperature

1 tablespoon freshly squeezed lemon juice

1 teaspoon pure vanilla extract

1 pound confectioners' sugar, sifted

Thin lemon slices, for garnish (optional)

Fresh blueberries, for garnish (optional)

Preheat the oven to 350°F. Butter and flour two 9-inch cake pans and line the bottoms with rounds of waxed paper.

To make the cake, sift the flour, cornstarch, baking powder, baking soda, and salt into a bowl and set aside. Place the butter in the bowl of an electric mixer and beat on medium-high speed until fluffy and light-colored. Gradually add the sugar, beating until well blended. Add the eggs 1 at a time, beating to fully incorporate each. Beat in the lemon juice, zest, and vanilla. Alternately add ¾ cup of the flour mixture and 1 tablespoon of the buttermilk until all is used. Fold in the berries and transfer the batter to the prepared cake pans. Bake for about 40 minutes, or

(continued)

until a toothpick inserted in the center of the cake comes out clean. If using frozen berries, extend the baking time by 5 to 8 minutes. Remove from the oven and let cool in the pans for 30 minutes. Invert onto a wire rack.

To make the frosting, using an electric mixer, beat the cream cheese and butter on medium-high speed until light and fluffy. Add the lemon juice and vanilla. Gradually add the confectioners' sugar and beat until smooth.

To assemble the cake, place 1 cake on a cake plate, bottom side facing up, and peel off the waxed paper. Top with 1½ cups of the frosting. Add the second cake, bottom side facing up, and peel off the waxed paper. Spread the remaining frosting on the sides and top. Refrigerate for at least 1 hour. Garnish with thin lemon slices or fresh blueberries.

Serves 12 to 16

Blueberry Spiced Doughnuts

Children of all ages love to make these special treats at home. Doughnuts require extra planning and more time than most recipes, but the results are well worth it.

¼ cup milk
¼ cup plus 1 teaspoon sugar
1 teaspoon active dry yeast
1½ cups all-purpose flour
⅛ teaspoon ground nutmeg
¼ teaspoon ground cinnamon
½ teaspoon salt
1 large egg
1 tablespoon water
2 tablespoons unsalted butter, melted
½ cup blueberries, chopped in food processor
Canola oil

Topping

½ cup sugar
1½ teaspoons ground cinnamon
⅛ teaspoon ground nutmeg
¼ teaspoon salt

(continued)

In a small saucepan, heat the milk over low heat until warm, not hot. Pour the milk into a small bowl and stir in 1 teaspoon of the sugar and the yeast. Let sit for 10 minutes, until the mixture is foamy. In the bowl of an electric mixer fitted with a paddle attachment, place the flour, the remaining ¼ cup sugar, the nutmeg, cinnamon, and salt. In a separate bowl, whisk together the egg and water. With the mixer on a low speed, add the yeast mixture, egg mixture, butter, and blueberries to the dry ingredients, mixing until just combined. Remove the paddle attachment and replace with a dough hook. On medium speed, mix with the dough hook for 20 minutes.

Oil a medium bowl. Transfer the dough from the mixer (it will be slightly sticky) to the bowl. Cover and refrigerate overnight.

Remove the dough from the refrigerator. On a lightly floured work surface, roll out the dough to ¼ inch thick. Cover in plastic wrap and return to the refrigerator for 30 minutes.

Meanwhile, combine all of the ingredients for the topping in a large bowl and set aside. Remove the dough from the refrigerator. Line a baking sheet with parchment paper and spray with vegetable oil cooking spray. With a doughnut cutter or the rim of a glass, cut the doughnuts into 1-inch circles and place on the parchment-lined baking sheet. Spray a second sheet of parchment and place on top of the doughnuts. Put the doughnuts in a warm place to rise for 30 minutes.

In a large heavy saucepan, heat 3 inches of canola oil over medium-high heat until very hot. Carefully drop the doughnuts into the oil in batches, being careful not to crowd them. Fry for 1 to 2 minutes on each side or until golden brown, turning them with tongs. Using a slotted spoon, transfer to a plate lined with paper towels. Continue frying a few at a time until all of the doughnuts are cooked. Toss with the topping and serve immediately.

Makes 2 dozen doughnuts

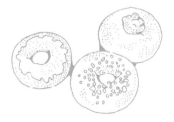

Blueberry Strudel

These luscious little strudels taste as good as a flaky pie without all the work. Serve them with cream on fine china or eat them with your fingers!

4½ cups fresh or unthawed frozen blueberries

⅔ cup sugar

3 tablespoons cornstarch

1 tablespoon freshly squeezed lemon juice

1 teaspoon pure almond extract

15 (17 by 12-inch) phyllo sheets, thawed

½ cup unsalted butter, melted

To make the filling, combine the blueberries, sugar, and cornstarch in a heavy saucepan over medium heat. Boil for 2 minutes. Remove from the heat and stir in the lemon juice. Let the filling cool for 10 minutes, then add the almond extract. You should have 2 cups of filling.

While the filling cools, arrange 3 sheets of phyllo side by side on a work surface to dry, about 15 minutes. Keeping the other 12 sheets stacked, cut them in half and stack the halves. Cover the dough with plastic wrap and a slightly damp kitchen towel to prevent the dough from drying out. Crumble the 3 dried sheets of dough and place in a small bowl.

Preheat the oven to 400°F. Grease a baking sheet with butter and set aside. Place 1 sheet of phyllo on the work surface with the short side facing you, and brush with melted butter. Place another sheet on top of this one and brush with butter. Continue until the stack contains 4 layers. Sprinkle about 2 tablespoons of the crumbled dried phyllo on the bottom third of the dough stack and top with ⅓ cup of the filling. Fold the short side up over the filling and fold up the sides. Roll the dough to form a strudel that measures 4½ by 2½ inches. Once rolled, brush all sides with melted butter. Transfer to the prepared baking sheet. Repeat this process with the remaining phyllo and filling to make strudels. Bake the strudels for 20 to 25 minutes, until crisp and light brown. Transfer to a wire rack to cool. Serve warm.

Makes 6 strudels

Blueberry-Peach Crisp

Take advantage of two favorite summer fruits in this tasty crisp. The topping is rich and crunchy, like an oatmeal cookie. Serve with whipped cream or vanilla ice cream.

3 cups fresh or partially thawed frozen blueberries

3 large peaches, pitted and sliced into wedges

⅔ cup granulated sugar

1½ teaspoons ground cinnamon

2 tablespoons quick-cooking tapioca

¾ cup plus 1 tablespoon all-purpose flour

1 cup instant oatmeal

¾ cup packed light brown sugar

⅛ teaspoon salt

½ cup unsalted butter, cold, cut into small pieces

½ cup chopped walnuts

Preheat the oven to 350°F. In a large bowl, mix together the blueberries, peaches, granulated sugar, cinnamon, tapioca, and 1 tablespoon of the flour. Let stand for 15 minutes.

Combine the remaining ¾ cup flour, the oatmeal, brown sugar, salt, and butter in a large bowl. Rub with your fingers until the butter is no longer distinguishable and the mixture resembles coarse crumbs. Stir in the walnuts. Place the fruit in a 1½ or 2-quart casserole dish and cover with the topping. Bake in the center of the oven for 50 minutes to 1 hour, until the fruit is tender and the topping is golden brown. Serve warm or at room temperature. Will keep covered in refrigerator for 3 days.

Serves 8 to 10

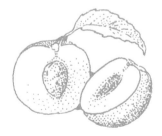

Classic Blueberry Pie

Blueberries contain five times more antioxidants than other fruits and vegetables. Consider a slice of this pie a healthy addition to your diet.

Pastry

2¼ cups all-purpose flour

½ teaspoon salt

1 tablespoon granulated sugar

½ cup unsalted butter, cold, cut into small pieces

⅓ cup shortening

6 tablespoons ice water

Filling

3 tablespoons all-purpose flour

1 tablespoon cornstarch

⅛ teaspoon salt

1 cup granulated sugar

1 tablespoon freshly squeezed lemon juice

½ teaspoon ground cinnamon

5 cups blueberries

2 tablespoons unsalted butter

To make the pastry, combine the flour, salt, and sugar in the bowl of a food processor fitted with the metal blade. Pulse to combine. Add the butter and shortening and pulse until the mixture resembles coarse meal. Add the ice water 1 tablespoon at a time, pulsing to incorporate. Continue until dough begins to pull together. Divide the dough into 2 balls, cover with plastic wrap, and refrigerate for 30 minutes.

Just before the dough is finished chilling, preheat the oven to 350°F. To make the filling, in a large bowl, combine the flour, cornstarch, salt, sugar, lemon juice, cinnamon, and blueberries. Set aside. On a lightly floured work surface, roll out the first ball of dough to ⅛ inch thick. Place the dough in an ungreased 9-inch deep-dish pie plate, allowing ¼ inch to hang over the edge. Spoon in the fruit mixture. Cut the butter into small pieces and dot the top of the fruit mixture with it. Roll out the second ball of

(continued)

dough to ⅛ inch thick. Cover the pie with the top crust, crimp the edges, and pierce the top with a knife to make vent holes.

To make the topping, in a small bowl, whisk together the egg and milk. Brush the egg mixture over the top of the pie and sprinkle with the turbinado sugar. Bake in the oven for 1 hour. The juices will be bubbling through the vent and the pastry will be nicely browned. Remove from the oven and let the pie cool for 30 minutes on a wire rack before cutting into slices to serve. Pie is best served same day but can be refrigerated up to 3 days.

Serves 8

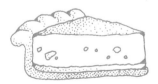